SBAs and EMQs in Obstetrics and Gynaecology for Medical Students

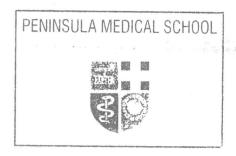

SBAs and EMQs in Obstetrics and Gynaecology for Medical Students

DR NEEL SHARMA

BSc (Hons), MBChB
Foundation Year Two Doctor
Homerton University Hospital NHS Foundation Trust
London

Foreword by
DR TIAGO VILLANUEVA
Past Editor of the *Student BMJ*

Radcliffe Publishing
Oxford • New York

Radcliffe Publishing Ltd
18 Marcham Road
Abingdon
Oxon OX14 1AA
United Kingdom

www.radcliffe-oxford.com

Electronic catalogue and worldwide online ordering facility.

British Library Cataloguing in Publication Data

A catalogue record for this book is available from the British Library.

ISBN-13: 978 184619 428 3

The paper used for the text pages of this book is FSC certified. FSC (The Forest Stewardship Council) is an international network to promote responsible management of the world's forests.

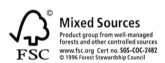

Mixed Sources
Product group from well-managed
forests and other controlled sources
www.fsc.org Cert no. SGS-COC-2482
© 1996 Forest Stewardship Council

Typeset by Pindar NZ, Auckland, New Zealand
Printed and bound by TJI Digital, Padstow, Cornwall, UK

Contents

Foreword

Are you frustrated with your slow and painstaking obstetrics and gynaecology revision? Are exams looming and are you becoming increasingly nervous? Well, Dr Neel Sharma's latest book may be the solution. It gives you hundreds of practice SBAs and EMQs on a very important field of medicine that for many of you is the staple content of undergraduate examinations. In addition, it allows you to review key concepts and fine tune your revision since the answer to every question is explained and commented on in concise detail. Regardless of your level of obstetrics and gynaecology knowledge and experience, this book will most definitely have something to offer you.

Dr Tiago Villanueva
Past Editor of the *Student BMJ*
November 2009

Preface

As a recent medical graduate I understand all too well the pressures faced during medical school. Lectures, tutorials, never-ending ward rounds, outpatient clinics, course work assignments and, of course, let us not forget the gruelling end-of-year exams. Trying to retain and, more importantly, understand all the common (and not-so-common) clinical diseases and presentations truly seems an impossible task.

With the advent of the Universities Medical Assessment Partnership (UMAP) there has now been a move away from testing specific clinical facts to an assessment focused on preparing yourself as a foundation doctor and the knowledge such a trainee needs on a daily basis. Currently, 14 UK medical schools are part of UMAP and their exams now require candidates to decide, for example, what would be the most appropriate initial investigation or what management plan they would instigate first when faced with a clinical problem. This is hardly an easy task based on the little experience one gains as an undergraduate in such decisions.

This self-assessment book is designed to help students tackle both the new form of assessment as well as the traditional style of examination. Questions covering all common obstetric and gynaecological presentations are included as SBA and EMQ formats with relevant, concise explanations as answers.

I sincerely hope that this book is of use in preparing for your forthcoming examinations and wish you all the success in your future medical careers.

Neel Sharma
November 2009

Education and work are the levers to uplift a people. Work alone will not do it unless inspired by the right ideals and guided by intelligence.

WEB Du Bois 1868–1963

I would like to dedicate this book to my parents, Ravi and Anita, and my sister Ravnita. Without their continued support and encouragement none of this would have truly been possible.

Useful references

American Journal of Obstetrics and Gynaecology. Available at: www.ajog.
org/

BJOG: An international journal of obstetrics and gynaecology. Available at:
www.bjog.org/view/0/index.html

Collins S, Arulkumaran S, Hayes K *et al. Oxford Handbook of Obstetrics
and Gynaecology*. Oxford: Oxford University Press; 2008.

The Royal College of Obstetricians and Gynaecologists. Available at:
www.rcog.org.uk

Questions

Single best answer

1 A middle-aged woman presents to her GP. She has been trying to get pregnant, but despite regular intercourse with her partner has been unable to do so. She enquires about when in her menstrual cycle she is likely to conceive. What is the most likely time frame in an average 28-day cycle when women are most likely to conceive?

a Day 2–4
b Day 4–6
c Day 8–10
d Day 8–14
e Day 16–20

2 The following are all common fetal complications associated with smoking in pregnancy EXCEPT:

a Prematurity
b Respiratory disease
c Intrauterine growth retardation
d Cot death
e Cystic fibrosis

3 The following are all common fetal complications associated with excessive alcohol consumption in pregnancy EXCEPT:

a Neurological damage

b Facial deformities

c Fetal growth retardation

d Increased birth weight

e Spontaneous miscarriage

4 A 32-year-old woman who is currently pregnant attends a routine antenatal care appointment. She enquires about the types of food she should avoid. She is requested to avoid eating large quantities of liver as it contains a vitamin strongly associated with congenital abnormalities. What is the vitamin most commonly associated with such abnormalities?

a Vitamin B

b Vitamin E

c Vitamin A

d Vitamin K

e Vitamin D

5 A 23-year-old recently pregnant woman attends a routine GP follow up appointment. The GP advises her to commence taking folic acid to reduce the risk of neural tube defects. What is the most commonly recommended dose of folic acid she should take?

a 100 micrograms

b 200 micrograms

c 300 micrograms

d 400 micrograms

e 500 micrograms

6   The following drugs should most definitely be avoided in pregnancy EXCEPT:

a   Paracetamol

b   Propranolol

c   Warfarin

d   Diclofenac

e   Furosemide

7   A 25-year-old recently pregnant woman presents to her GP. She is keen to know the risk of her baby having Down's syndrome. The GP explains the possibility of having a triple test. What are the most common serum markers that comprise the triple test?

a   Beta human chorionic gonadotropin (βhCG), estriol, alpha-fetoprotein (AFP)

b   Alpha-fetoprotein (AFP), inhibin A, pregnancy-associated plasma protein A (PAPP A)

c   Estriol, alpha-fetoprotein (AFP), inhibin A

d   Beta human chorionic gonadotropin (βhCG), alpha-fetoprotein (AFP), inhibin A

e   Pregnancy-associated plasma protein A (PAPP A), alpha-fetoprotein (AFP), estriol

8 A 26-year-old recently pregnant woman presents to her GP. She is keen to know the risk of her baby having Down's syndrome. The GP explains the possibility of having an ultrasound scan. What is the most appropriate time frame for performing such a scan?

a 2–4 weeks gestation

b 4–6 weeks gestation

c 8–10 weeks gestation

d 11–14 weeks gestation

e 14–18 weeks gestation

9 A 26-year-old recently pregnant woman presents to her GP. She is keen to know whether her baby has Down's syndrome. The GP explains the possibility of an amniocentesis. What is the most appropriate time frame for performing such a procedure?

a 6 weeks gestation

b 8 weeks gestation

c 10 weeks gestation

d 12 weeks gestation

e 15 weeks gestation

10 A recently pregnant woman is keen to undergo amniocentesis to determine whether her baby has Down's syndrome. You explain the procedure and inform her that there is a risk of miscarriage. What is the most likely percentage risk of a miscarriage?

a 1%

b 2%

c 3%

d 4%

e 5%

11 A recently pregnant woman presents to her GP wanting to know if her baby has Down's syndrome. Her GP refers her for chorionic villous sampling. What is the most appropriate time frame for such an investigation?

a 6–8 weeks gestation

b 8–10 weeks gestation

c 11–14 weeks gestation

d 16–18 weeks gestation

e 18–20 weeks gestation

12 A middle-aged woman who is currently 12 weeks pregnant is referred for a routine ultrasound scan. The following are all commonly detected at this time EXCEPT:

a Anencephaly

b Oligohydramnios

c Cystic hydroma

d Bladder outflow obstruction

e Abdominal wall defects

13 A middle-aged woman attends her 25-week antenatal care appointment. The following are all commonly assessed at this time EXCEPT:

a Blood pressure

b Urine

c Symphysis fundal height (SFH)

d Fetal heart beat

e Fetal position

14 The following physiological changes occur during pregnancy EXCEPT:

    a A fall in blood pressure in early pregnancy

    b An increase in maternal ventilation

    c Hypercoagulability

    d An increase in the glomerular filtration rate

    e An increase in gastric emptying

15 A middle-aged pregnant women presents to her GP complaining of feeling nauseous and vomiting up to four times a week. What is the most likely aetiological cause for her symptoms?

    a Prolactin

    b Progesterone

    c Oestrogen

    d βhCG

    e AFP

16 The following serum markers increase during pregnancy EXCEPT:

    a T3

    b Protein

    c Alkaline phosphatase

    d T4

    e Thyroxine-binding globulin (TBG)

17 A middle-aged pregnant woman presents to her GP complaining of a sudden onset headache and visual disturbance. She has no known past medical history. On examination you note her blood pressure is 145/90 mm Hg. She has evidence of epigastric tenderness and facial swelling. Urine dipstick confirms 1+ protein. What is the most likely diagnosis?

a Nephrotic syndrome

b Pre-eclampsia

c Protein deficiency

d Hypothyroidism

e None of the above

18 A middle-aged pregnant woman is recently diagnosed with pre-eclampsia. The following are all risk factors for pre-eclampsia EXCEPT:

a Diabetes

b Hypertension

c Renal disease

d Molar pregnancy

e Anorexia

19 The following serum markers all rise in pre-eclampsia EXCEPT:

a Platelets

b Urea

c Creatinine

d Aspartate aminotransferase (AST)

e Alanine aminotransferase (ALT)

20 A 32-year-old pregnant woman has been recently diagnosed with pre-eclampsia. Routine observations reveal a blood pressure of 145/90 mm Hg. Which management plan would you instigate first to help control her blood pressure?

    a Labetalol

    b Nifedipine

    c Methyldopa

    d Hydralazine

    e Ramipril

21 A 31-year-old woman who is currently 38 weeks pregnant has been recently diagnosed with pre-eclampsia. Routine observations reveal a blood pressure of 150/90 mm Hg. On examination you note evidence of epigastric tenderness. A recent full blood count reveals a haemoglobin of 8.4 g/dL, a white cell count of 10×10^9/L and a platelet count of 98×10^9/L. What is the next most appropriate step in management?

    a Labetalol

    b Immediate delivery

    c Nifedipine

    d Continue to observe

    e Ramipril

22 The following are all common complications of pre-eclampsia EXCEPT:

a Pulmonary oedema

b Disseminated intravascular coagulation (DIC)

c Cerebral haemorrhage

d Eclampsia

e Placenta praevia

23 A 25-year-old woman who is currently 28 weeks pregnant presents to A&E following an episode of vaginal bleeding. She denies any abdominal pain or discomfort. On examination you note fresh red blood. What is the most likely diagnosis?

a Placenta praevia

b Placental abruption

c Vasa praevia

d Infection

e Malignancy

24 A 26-year-old woman who is currently 29 weeks pregnant presents to A&E following an episode of vaginal bleeding. She complains of severe abdominal pain. On examination you note dark red blood. Abdominal palpation reveals a hard 'woody' uterus. What is the most likely diagnosis?

a Placenta praevia

b Placental abruption

c Vasa praevia

d Infection

e Malignancy

25 A 26-year-old woman who is currently 30 weeks pregnant presents to A&E following an episode of vaginal bleeding. She denies any abdominal pain or discomfort. On examination you note evidence of a high fetal head. What is the most likely diagnosis?

a Placenta praevia

b Placental abruption

c Vasa praevia

d Infection

e Malignancy

26 A 26-year-old woman who is currently 30 weeks pregnant presents to A&E following an episode of vaginal bleeding. On examination you note fresh red blood. What is the next most appropriate initial investigation?

a Vaginal swab

b Abdominal ultrasound scan

c Abdominal X-ray

d Pelvic X-ray

e Abdominal CT scan

27 A 32-year-old woman presents to A&E following an episode of heavy vaginal bleeding. She is currently 29 weeks pregnant. She complains of severe abdominal pain. Routine observations reveal a blood pressure of 90/50 mm Hg and pulse rate of 140 beats per minute. She is pale in appearance and clammy to touch. What is the next most appropriate step in management?

a Vaginal swab

b Abdominal ultrasound scan

c Cardiotocography

d Abdominal X-ray

e IV access and urgent fluid resuscitation

28 The following are all risk factors for placental abruption EXCEPT:

a Hypertension

b Pre-eclampsia

c Diabetes

d Alcohol

e Tobacco use

29 A 29-year-old woman who is currently 37 weeks pregnant presents to A&E following an episode of fresh red vaginal bleeding. She denies any abdominal pain or discomfort. Routine observations reveal a blood pressure of 125/80 mm Hg and pulse rate of 85 beats per minute. Which management plan would you instigate first?

a Delivery by caesarean section

b Continue to observe

c IV access and blood product transfusion

d Abdominal CT scan

e Abdominal X-ray

30 According to the World Health Organization (WHO), which of the following criteria most appropriately diagnoses gestational diabetes mellitus?

a Two-hour venous glucose <7.8 mmol/L

b Two-hour venous glucose 7.8–11 mmol/L

c Two-hour venous glucose >11 mmol/L

d Two-hour venous glucose >10 mmol/L

e Two-hour venous glucose 10–11 mmol/L

31 The following are all associated risks in a diabetic pregnancy EXCEPT:

a Miscarriage

b Shoulder dystocia

c Infection

d Oligohydramnios

e Cord prolapse

32 A 25-year-old woman presents to her GP. She is currently in her second trimester of pregnancy. She complains of severe itching of her legs and arms. There is no evidence of a rash on examination. The GP is concerned about cholestasis and arranges urgent liver function tests. The following are all complications in pregnancy associated with cholestasis EXCEPT:

a Fetal distress

b Pre-term delivery

c Intrauterine death

d Intracranial fetal haemorrhage

e Shoulder dystocia

33 A 36-week pregnant woman presents to her GP for a routine check up. On examination you palpate the head in the fundus of the uterus and in the midline. What is the most likely diagnosis?

a Footling breech

b Extended breech

c Flexed breech

d Multiple pregnancy

e None of the above

34 A 36-week pregnant woman presents to her GP for a check up. On examination you palpate the head in the fundus of the uterus. What is the next most appropriate step in management?

a External cephalic version

b Continue to observe

c Immediate caesarean section

d Induced vaginal delivery

e Abdominal CT scan

35 The following are all risk factors for multiple pregnancy EXCEPT:

a Positive family history

b Assisted conception

c Increasing parity

d Obesity

e Young maternal age

36 The following are all common maternal complications of multiple pregnancy EXCEPT:

a Miscarriage

b Renal failure

c Gestational diabetes

d Placental praevia

e Anaemia

37 The following are all common fetal complications of multiple pregnancy EXCEPT:

a Pre-term labour

b Intrauterine growth retardation

c Malpresentation

d Jaundice

e Shoulder dystocia

38 The following are all true with regards to labour EXCEPT:

a Labour typically occurs between the 37th and 42nd week of pregnancy

b The second stage of labour is associated with dilatation of the cervix

c The third stage of labour is the interval between delivery of the fetus to delivery of the placenta

d The cervix is drawn up into the lower uterine segment

e It is associated with the passage of a mucus plug

39 The following statements are all true with regards to labour EXCEPT:

a Engagement is defined as less than or equal to two-fifths of the fetal head palpable above the pelvic brim

b In maximum flexion the posterior fontanelle can be palpated vaginally

c Internal rotation involves rotation of the fetal head from the occipito transverse to the left occipital transverse position

d Restitution is where the fetal head reverts to the transverse position

e Descent tends to occur just before the onset of labour in Afro-Caribbean women

40 The following are all true with regards to the progress of labour in primiparous patients EXCEPT:

a The cervix dilates typically 1 cm per hour

b The second stage of labour lasts for 2 hours

c The first stage of labour lasts for 10 hours

d The uterus is prone to rupture

e Labour lasting longer than 12 hours is classified as prolonged

41 The following are all true with regards to fetal surveillance in labour EXCEPT:

a The absence of liquor is associated with intrauterine growth retardation

b Auscultation with a pinard stethoscope should occur every five minutes

c A fetal blood pH of greater than 7.25 is normal

d The passage of meconium signifies hypoxia

e A fetal blood pH of less than 7.2 indicates immediate delivery

42 The following are all true with regards to fetal heart rate EXCEPT:

a A tachycardia is greater than 160 beats per minute

b A bradycardia is less than 80 beats per minute

c Early decelerations occur with the onset of a contraction

d A tachycardia may be due to hypoxia

e A bradycardia may be due to hypoxia

43 The following are all true with regards to the third stage of labour EXCEPT:

a Syntometrine is given to all women in labour

b Cord clamping takes place when cord pulsation has stopped

c Syntometrine is given intramuscularly

d The placenta is removed manually after an hour has elapsed

e Cord traction is performed

44   The following are all indications for labour induction EXCEPT:

   a   Antepartum haemorrhage

   b   Intrauterine growth retardation

   c   Maternal hypertension

   d   Post-maturity

   e   Bacterial vaginosis

45   A 25-year-old woman presents to A&E. She is currently 41 weeks
     pregnant. She is referred to the obstetric registrar on call who
     feels she is a candidate for immediate surgical induction of labour.
     What is the most appropriate Bishop's score required prior to such
     induction?

   a   1

   b   2

   c   4

   d   5

   e   7 and above

46   A 28-year-old woman presents to A&E in labour. She is referred
     immediately to the obstetrician on call. It is noted that the second
     stage is prolonged after one hour of active maternal pushing. The
     obstetrician decides to expedite delivery with forceps. The follow-
     ing are all important criteria prior to commencement of operative
     delivery EXCEPT:

   a   Full dilation of the cervix

   b   Ruptured membranes

   c   A full maternal bladder

   d   No excessive moulding

   e   Adequate analgesia

47 A middle-aged woman presents to A&E in labour. She is referred to the obstetrician on call. It is noted that the second stage is prolonged after one hour of active maternal pushing. The obstetrician decides to expedite delivery with ventouse suction. The following are all true with regards to ventouse delivery EXCEPT:

a The procedure should be performed with the patient in the lithotomy position

b Traction should take place during uterine contractions

c A maximal force should be applied

d An episiotomy may be required

e Adequate analgesia is required

48 A 32-year-old woman presents to A&E in labour. You note a cervical diameter of 5 cm after seven hours. Which management plan would you instigate first?

a Ventouse delivery

b Forceps delivery

c Prostaglandin pessaries

d Oxytocin IV

e Caesarean section

49 The following are all true with regards to pre-term labour EXCEPT:

a The fetus is typically delivered between 24 and 37 weeks of pregnancy

b Salbutamol promotes fetal lung maturity

c It is often the result of pre-eclampsia

d It is often the result of polyhydramnios

e It is often associated with trichomonas infection

50 A middle-aged woman is three weeks post-delivery. She presents to her GP complaining of swelling and pain in her right breast. On examination there is evidence of erythema and moderate tenderness. Routine observations reveal a temperature of 38.5°C. What is the most likely aetiological cause for such a presentation?

a *Staphylococcus aureus*

b *Escherichia coli*

c *Klebsiella*

d *Mycobacterium tuberculosis*

e *Haemophilus influenzae*

51 Which management plan would you instigate first in the above patient?

a Trimethoprim

b Flucloxacillin

c Paracetamol

d Encourage oral fluids

e Rifampicin

52 A 24-year-old woman presents to A&E following an episode of heavy vaginal bleeding. She is currently two weeks post-delivery. Routine observations reveal a blood pressure of 90/50 mm Hg and pulse rate of 140 beats per minute. Speculum examination reveals an open cervical os. Bimanual examination reveals a soft bulky uterus. What is the most likely diagnosis?

    a Retained products of conception

    b Endometritis

    c Placenta praevia

    d Placental abruption

    e Menorrhagia

53 Which investigation is most likely to lead to a diagnosis in the above patient?

    a Vaginal swab

    b Full blood count

    c Abdominal CT scan

    d Transvaginal ultrasound scan

    e C reactive protein

54 A 26-year-old woman has just given birth. Her newborn baby undergoes assessment. He is pink in appearance and has a heart rate of 125 beats per minute. He demonstrates a strong respiratory effort, good flexion and coughs when stimulated. What is the most likely Apgar score?

a 2

b 4

c 6

d 8

e 10

55 A middle-aged woman is in active labour. The head has been delivered slowly, but the neck does not appear with the chin retracting against the perineum. What is the most likely diagnosis?

a Uterine rupture

b Uterine inversion

c Placenta praevia

d Shoulder dystocia

e Cord prolapse

56 The following are all risk factors for the above presentation EXCEPT:

a Slow progress in the first stage

b Slow progress in the second stage

c Macrosomia

d Post-maturity

e An underweight mother

57 The following are all true with regards to primary post-partum haemorrhage EXCEPT:

a It is associated with greater than 500 mL blood loss within the first 24 hours post-delivery

b It can be due to uterine atony

c It can be due to vaginal lacerations

d It is associated with oligohydramnios

e It is associated with prolonged labour

58 A 24-year-old woman presents to her GP. She is keen to start some form of contraceptive as she is currently sexually active. She is known to suffer from heavy periods. She is a non-smoker and non-drinker. What is the next most appropriate step in management?

a Progesterone-only pill

b Combined oral contraceptive pill

c The diaphragm

d The coil

e The implant device

59 A 36-year-old woman presents to her GP. She is keen to start some form of contraceptive as she is in an active sexual relationship. She is a heavy smoker and drinker. She is known to suffer from migraines. Which of the following is specifically contraindicated in terms of contraception?

a Progesterone-only pill

b Combined oral contraceptive pill

c The diaphragm

d The coil

e The implant device

60   A middle-aged woman is currently on the combined oral contra-
      ceptive pill. She presents to her GP stating that she has missed one
      of her pills. She is currently sexually active. What is the next most
      appropriate step in management?

      a Reassure

      b Resume the pack as normal

      c Resume the pack as normal and use a barrier method of
         contraception for seven days

      d Commence the progesterone-only pill

      e Utilise a barrier method of contraception for the next
         48 hours

61   A 35-year-old woman presents to her GP. She is in an active sexual
      relationship and is keen to commence some form of contraception.
      She is a life-long smoker and has a history of hypertension. She has
      suffered from pelvic inflammatory disease in the past. There is a
      family history of endometrial cancer. What is the next most appro-
      priate step in management?

      a Progesterone-only pill

      b Combined oral contraceptive pill

      c The diaphragm

      d The copper coil

      e The implant device

62 A 31-year-old woman presents to her GP. She complains of a new onset headache and weight gain. Routine observations reveal a blood pressure of 160/40 mm Hg. She has recently been started on a new contraceptive device. What is the most likely aetiological cause for her symptoms?

a Progesterone-only pill

b Combined oral contraceptive pill

c The diaphragm

d The coil

e The implant device

63 A middle-aged woman presents to her GP. She is keen to commence some form of contraception. She has a past medical history of hypertension for which she takes ramipril and she has been treated for pelvic inflammatory disease in the past. She comments that she is getting forgetful and has difficulty in remembering to take her tablets. What is the next most appropriate step in management?

a Progesterone-only pill

b Combined oral contraceptive pill

c The diaphragm

d The cap

e The implant device

64 A 45-year-old woman presents to her GP. She is keen to commence some form of contraception. She has recently been diagnosed with osteoporosis. She is a non-smoker and non-drinker. The following are all suitable forms of contraception EXCEPT:

a Progesterone-only pill

b Combined oral contraceptive pill

c The diaphragm

d Medroxyprogesterone IM

e The implant device

65 A 31-year-old woman presents to her GP seeking contraception. She is known to have had an ectopic pregnancy in the past. She is a light smoker and occasional drinker. What is the next most appropriate step in management?

a Progesterone-only pill

b Combined oral contraceptive pill

c The diaphragm

d Medroxyprogesterone IM

e Mirena coil

66 A 26-year-old woman presents to her GP requesting a suitable form of contraception. She has a history of menorrhagia and pelvic inflammatory disease. Which of the following is the least suitable form of contraception?

a Progesterone-only pill

b Combined oral contraceptive pill

c Copper coil

d Medroxyprogesterone IM

e Mirena coil

67 The following are all true with regards to emergency contraception EXCEPT:

   a A copper intrauterine contraceptive device must be inserted within 72 hours of unprotected intercourse

   b The levonorgestrel pill is recommended at a dose of 5 mg

   c The side-effects of levonorgestrel include irregular bleeding

   d The levonorgestrel pill works via inhibition of egg transport

   e The copper intrauterine contraceptive device prevents at least 98% of expected pregnancies

68 A middle-aged woman presents to her GP following an episode of unprotected intercourse. She complains of lower abdominal pain, a pus-like discharge and irregular bleeding. The GP is concerned about the possibility of *Neisseria gonorrhoeae*. Which investigation is most likely to lead to a diagnosis?

   a Endocervical swab

   b Vaginal swab

   c Abdominal ultrasound scan

   d Abdominal CT scan

   e Blood cultures

69 A 23-year-old woman presents to her GP. She complains of lower abdominal pain and irregular vaginal bleeding. She admits to having an episode of unprotected intercourse recently. An endocervical swab confirms the diagnosis as chlamydia. Which management plan would you instigate first?

a Azithromycin

b Continue to observe

c Procaine penicillin

d Ciprofloxacin

e Metronidazole

70 A 25-year-old woman presents to her GP following an episode of unprotected intercourse. She complains of a foul smelling yellow vaginal discharge and dysuria. On examination you note evidence of a strawberry-red cervix. What is the most likely diagnosis?

a Chlamydia

b Genital herpes

c Trichomonas

d *Neisseria gonorrhoeae*

e Syphilis

71 What is the next most appropriate step in management with regards to the above patient?

a Azithromycin

b Doxycycline

c Procaine penicillin

d Ciprofloxacin

e Metronidazole

72 A middle-aged woman presents to her GP following an episode of unprotected intercourse. She complains of the presence of several small labial blisters and feeling generally unwell. Which investigation is most likely to lead to a diagnosis?

    a Abdominal ultrasound scan

    b Pelvic ultrasound scan

    c Transvaginal ultrasound scan

    d Endocervical swab

    e Lesion swab

73 A middle-aged woman presents to her GP following an episode of unprotected intercourse. On examination you note the presence of several small labial blisters. Which management plan would you instigate first?

    a Azithromycin

    b Doxycycline

    c Aciclovir

    d Ciprofloxacin

    e Metronidazole

74 A 35-year-old woman presents to A&E. She has recently had an episode of unprotected intercourse. On examination you note the presence of several pedunculated lesions on her vagina approximately 5 mm in size. Which management plan would you instigate first?

    a Podophyllin

    b Doxycycline

    c Aciclovir

    d Ciprofloxacin

    e Metronidazole

75 A 23-year-old escort presents to A&E. She complains of the presence of a single ulcer on her genitalia. She denies any pain or discomfort. What is the most likely diagnosis?

a Primary syphilis

b Secondary syphilis

c Latent syphilis

d Tertiary syphilis

e Congenital syphilis

76 What is the most likely aetiological agent responsible for the above patient's presentation?

a *Neisseria gonorrhoeae*

b *Treponema pallidum*

c *Chlamydia trachomatis*

d *Staphylococcus aureus*

e *Haemophilus influenzae*

77 A 35-year-old married woman presents to her GP. She complains of feeling unwell with non-specific joint pains and perianal discomfort. On examination you note evidence of wart like lesions on her perineum. She admits to being unfaithful to her husband for several years. What is the most likely diagnosis?

a Primary syphilis

b Secondary syphilis

c Latent syphilis

d Tertiary syphilis

e Congenital syphilis

78 A middle-aged woman presents to her GP following an episode of unprotected intercourse. She complains of a single painless ulcer within her vagina. What is the next most appropriate step in management?

a Podophyllin

b Flucloxacillin

c Aciclovir

d Ciprofloxacin

e Procaine penicillin

79 A 24-year-old woman presents to A&E following an episode of unprotected intercourse. She complains of generalised abdominal pain and irregular bleeding. Speculum examination reveals evidence of a discharge. Bimanual examination demonstrates evidence of cervical excitation. What is the most likely aetiological cause for such symptoms?

a *Neisseria gonorrhoeae*

b *Treponema pallidum*

c *Chlamydia trachomatis*

d *Gardnerella vaginalis*

e *Haemophilus influenzae*

80 A middle-aged woman presents to her GP. She complains of a grey curd-like vaginal discharge. She has a past medical history of type II diabetes. What is the most likely diagnosis?

a Candida

b Genital herpes

c Trichomonas

d *Neisseria gonorrhoea*

e Syphilis

81 Which management plan would you instigate first in the above patient?

a Clotrimazole

b Flucloxacillin

c Aciclovir

d Ciprofloxacin

e Procaine penicillin

82 A middle-aged woman presents to her GP complaining of a cream-coloured discharge. She has had unprotected intercourse in the recent past. Microscopy reveals the presence of clue cells. What is the most likely diagnosis?

a Candida

b Genital herpes

c Trichomonas

d Bacterial vaginosis

e Syphilis

83 A middle-aged woman is recently diagnosed with Bacterial vaginosis. What is the most likely aetiological cause?

a *Neisseria gonorrhoeae*

b *Haemophilus influenzae*

c *Chlamydia trachomatis*

d *Staphylococcus aureus*

e *Gardnerella vaginalis*

84 A middle-aged pregnant woman is recently diagnosed with chlamydia. The following are all complications of chlamydial infection
EXCEPT:

a Pelvic inflammatory disease

b Ectopic pregnancy

c Infertility

d Pre-term delivery

e Macrosomia

85 A 23-year-old woman is recently diagnosed with *Neisseria gonorrhoea*.
According to gram staining, what is the most accurate classification
of this bacterium?

a Gram negative *coccus*

b Gram positive *coccus*

c Gram positive *rod*

d Gram positive *bacillus*

e Gram negative *diplococcus*

86 A 24-year-old woman presents to her GP complaining of a grey curd like vaginal discharge. Which investigation is most likely to lead to a diagnosis?

a High vaginal swab

b Endocervical swab

c Urethral swab

d Abdominal ultrasound scan

e Blood cultures

87 A 26-year-old woman presents to her GP following an episode of unprotected intercourse. She is concerned about the development of new lesions vaginally. On examination you note the presence of several pearl-white lesions approximately 5 mm in diameter. What is the most likely diagnosis?

a Molluscum contagiosum

b Genital herpes

c Trichomonas

d *Neisseria gonorrhoea*

e Syphilis

88 A 28-year-old woman presents to her GP complaining of new onset vaginal itching. She comments she has noted brown specks in her underwear. On further questioning she admits to having episodes of unprotected intercourse. What is the most likely diagnosis?

a Molluscum contagiosum

b Genital herpes

c Trichomonas

d Crabs

e Syphilis

89 A middle-aged woman is recently diagnosed with Bacterial vaginosis. The following are all true with regard to the diagnostic criteria for Bacterial vaginosis EXCEPT:

  a It is associated with a cream-coloured discharge

  b Clue cells are noted on microscopy

  c A fish-like odour is produced on the addition of potassium hydroxide to the discharge

  d It is associated with a vaginal fluid pH greater than 4.5

  e It is associated with irregular bleeding

90 According to the Pearl index what is the most effective form of contraception from the below list?

  a Male sterilization

  b Combined oral contraceptive pill

  c Female condom

  d Male condom

  e Progestogen implants

91 The following are all side-effects of the combined oral contraceptive pill EXCEPT:

  a Hypertension

  b Thrombosis

  c Migraine

  d Menorrhagia

  e Irregular bleeding

92 The following are all common side-effects of the progesterone-only pill EXCEPT:

a Ovarian cysts

b Weight loss

c Breast tenderness

d Headaches

e Nausea

93 The following are all common contraindications to the use of the Mirena coil EXCEPT:

a Pregnancy

b Liver failure

c Renal failure

d Mechanical heart valve

e Ovarian carcinoma

94 The following are all common contraindications to the use of the copper coil EXCEPT:

a Pregnancy

b Irregular bleeding

c Anaemia

d Wilson's disease

e Jaundice

95 A 53-year-old gentleman presents to his GP. He is keen to have a vasectomy but would like to know about the possible risks and complications. The following are all associated with a vasectomy EXCEPT:

a Failure

b Infection

c Sperm granuloma

d Malignancy

e Haematoma

96 A 34-year-old woman presents to her GP. She is currently 21 weeks pregnant. She complains of lower abdominal pain and heavy vaginal bleeding. Speculum examination reveals an open cervical os. There are no associated products of conception. What is the most likely diagnosis?

a Complete miscarriage

b Missed miscarriage

c Septic miscarriage

d Inevitable miscarriage

e Threatened miscarriage

97 A 28-year-old woman presents to A&E. She is currently 23 weeks pregnant. She complains of lower abdominal pain and vaginal bleeding. Speculum examination reveals no evidence of cervical dilatation. What is the most likely diagnosis?

a Complete miscarriage

b Missed miscarriage

c Septic miscarriage

d Inevitable miscarriage

e Threatened miscarriage

98 A 32-year-old woman presents to A&E. She is currently 14 weeks pregnant. She complains of lower abdominal pain and vaginal bleeding. Speculum examination reveals an open cervical os. You are concerned about the possibility of miscarriage. Which investigation is most likely to lead to a diagnosis?

a Abdominal CT scan

b Transvaginal ultrasound scan

c Full blood count

d Vaginal swab

e Abdominal X-ray

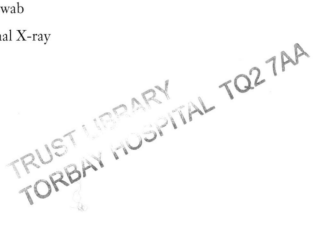

99 A 23-year-old woman presents to her GP. She is currently nine weeks pregnant. She is requesting an immediate termination as her partner is threatening to leave her if she goes ahead with the pregnancy. She is notably low in mood and threatening to self-harm. She has a fear of anaesthetic medication. What is the next most appropriate step in management?

a Suction curettage

b Antiprogesterone tablets with prostaglandin pessaries

c Dilatation of the cervix and evacuation of the uterine contents

d Prostaglandin induction

e Copper coil

100 According to the 1967 Abortion Act, the following are all indications for termination of pregnancy if pregnancy were to continue EXCEPT:

a The women's life is likely to be endangered

b The women's physical health is likely to be endangered

c The women's mental health is likely to be endangered

d The partner's physical health is likely to be endangered

e The child is likely to suffer a physical handicap

101 A 40-year-old woman presents to A&E. She is currently 10 weeks pregnant. She complains of lower abdominal pain and vaginal bleeding. She has had three miscarriages in the past. You are concerned about the possibility of a further miscarriage. What is the most likely aetiological cause if this were true?

a Fibroids

b Polycystic ovaries

c Antiphospholipid syndrome

d Bacterial vaginosis

e Cervical incompetence

102 A middle-aged woman who is currently pregnant presents to A&E. She complains of lower abdominal pain and irregular bleeding. Serum βhCG is 1600 IU. What is the most likely diagnosis?

a Complete miscarriage

b Missed miscarriage

c Septic miscarriage

d Ectopic pregnancy

e Threatened miscarriage

103 A 32-year-old woman who is currently pregnant presents to A&E. She complains of lower abdominal pain and irregular bleeding. You are concerned about the possibility of an ectopic pregnancy. Which investigation is most likely to lead to a diagnosis?

a Serum βhCG alone

b Abdominal CT scan

c Serum βhCG and transvaginal ultrasound scan

d Abdominal X-ray

e Vaginal swab

104 Which of the following is the most likely site of implantation in an ectopic pregnancy?

a Ovary

b Cervix

c Uterus

d Abdominal cavity

e Fallopian tube

105 A 34-year-old woman who is currently pregnant presents to A&E. She complains of lower abdominal pain and irregular bleeding. You are concerned about the possibility of an ectopic pregnancy. She has a past history of pelvic inflammatory disease and currently has a Mirena coil *in situ*. She was previously on the progesterone-only pill. What is the most likely aetiological cause for her possible ectopic?

a Mirena coil

b Pelvic inflammatory disease history

c Age

d The progesterone-only pill

e None of the above

106 With regards to the menstrual cycle, where is the gonadotropin-releasing hormone (GnRH) released from?

a The anterior pituitary gland

b The posterior pituitary gland

c The thyroid gland

d The adrenal gland

e The hypothalamus

107 The main hormone responsible for the ovulatory phase of the menstrual cycle is?

a Follicle-stimulating hormone (FSH)

b Luteinising hormone (LH)

c GnRH

d Thyroid-stimulating hormone (TSH)

e Progesterone

108 During the luteal phase of the menstrual cycle the corpus luteum produces which of the following hormones?

a FSH

b LH

c GnRH

d Progesterone alone

e Oestrogen and progesterone

109 Which of the following hormones is responsible for the growth and thickening of the endometrium?

a FSH

b LH

c GnRH

d Oestrogen

e Progesterone

110 Which of the following hormones is responsible for the vascularisation of the endometrium?

a FSH

b LH

c GnRH

d Oestrogen and Progesterone

e Progesterone alone

111 The following are all true with regards to the menstrual cycle EXCEPT:

a Menstruation is associated with endometrial necrosis

b Bleeding lasts for 3–5 days

c The length of the average cycle is 28 days

d The average loss of blood is 50–60 mL

e Menarche usually begins between the age of 11 and 15 years

112 A reduction in which of the following hormones is a trigger to the start of menstruation?

a FSH

b LH

c GnRH

d Oestrogen and progesterone

e Progesterone alone

113 A 25-year-old woman presents to her GP complaining of unusually heavy periods. She comments that she uses at least eight pads per day when she is on her period. Routine blood investigations confirm a haemoglobin of 8.2 g/dL. You arrange a set of haematinics and request a blood film. What is most likely to be noted on the blood film?

a Pencil cells

b Hypersegmented neutrophils

c Pancytopenia

d Sickle cells

e None of the above

114 A middle-aged woman presents to her GP complaining of unusually heavy periods. She comments that she has noticed clots of blood being passed as well. She is a heavy smoker and has a past medical history of hypertension. What is the next most appropriate step in management?

a Reassure

b Combined oral contraceptive pill

c Mefenamic acid

d Mirena coil

e Endometrial ablation

115 A middle-aged woman was diagnosed with menorrhagia by her GP approximately two months ago. She was started on appropriate therapy but has suffered from irregular bleeding ever since treatment was commenced. What treatment was she most likely to have started?

 a Progesterone-only pill

 b Combined oral contraceptive pill

 c Mefenamic acid

 d Mirena coil

 e Endometrial ablation

116 A middle-aged woman has been recently diagnosed with menorrhagia by her GP. She has been trialled on mefenamic acid and the Mirena coil, which failed to improve her symptoms. Her GP refers her for transcervical resection of the endometrium. The following are all common complications associated with this procedure EXCEPT:

 a Uterine perforation

 b Infection

 c Bleeding

 d Pregnancy

 e Malignancy

117 A 43-year-old woman presents to her GP. She complains of sudden onset pelvic pain, which occurs approximately two to three days prior to her period. She comments that the pain improves typically within the first day of bleeding. What is the next most appropriate step in management?

a Heat therapy

b Mefenamic acid

c Transcutaneous electrical nerve stimulation (TENS)

d Acupuncture

e Fentanyl patch

118 A 16-year-old girl presents to her GP. She is concerned that she has not as yet commenced her periods. On examination you note evidence of a webbed neck and short stature. What is the most likely diagnosis?

a Turner's syndrome

b Marfan's syndrome

c Huntington's chorea

d Noonan syndrome

e None of the above

119 A middle-aged woman is brought to her GP by her partner. He complains that she often becomes excessively irritable and tearful as she approaches her period. He comments that this has been the case for the past five years and he feels it is affecting their relationship. What is the next most appropriate step in management?

   a Olanzapine

   b Imipramine

   c Paracetamol

   d Fluoxetine

   e Risperidone

120 A middle-aged woman who is currently pregnant presents to A&E. She complains of lower abdominal pain and irregular bleeding. Routine observations reveal a pulse rate of 140 beats per minute and a blood pressure of 90/40 mm Hg. What is the next most appropriate step in management?

   a Transvaginal ultrasound scan

   b Abdominal CT scan

   c Urgent laparoscopy

   d Reassure

   e Methotrexate

121 A 35-year-old woman presents to her GP. She complains of irregular periods and acne predominantly on her face. What is the most likely diagnosis?

a Polycystic ovarian syndrome

b Endometriosis

c Cervical cancer

d Fibroids

e Kallman's syndrome

122 A middle-aged woman presents to her GP. She comments that her periods have stopped. On examination you note evidence of excessive hair growth on her chin. Which investigation is most likely to lead to a diagnosis?

a Urethral swab

b Abdominal X-ray

c Pelvic X-ray

d Abdominal ultrasound scan

e Vaginal swab

123 A middle-aged woman presents to her GP. She comments that her periods are irregular and that she has noticed her trousers and skirts feel tighter than normal. What is the next most appropriate initial investigation?

a Progesterone

b Thyroid function tests

c Prolactin

d LH:FSH ratio

e Oestrogen

124 A middle-aged woman presents to her GP. She comments that her periods are irregular and that her skin feels greasier than normal. On examination you note evidence of facial acne and hirsutism. What is the next most appropriate step in management?

    a Progesterone-only pill

    b Clearasil®

    c Combined oral contraceptive pill

    d Flucloxacillin

    e Reassure

125 A 25-year-old woman is recently diagnosed with polycystic ovarian syndrome. The following are all likely investigative findings EXCEPT:

    a Raised testosterone

    b Decreased sex hormone binding globulin

    c Raised FSH

    d Raised LH

    e Normal thyroid function tests

126 The following are all likely complications of polycystic ovarian syndrome EXCEPT:

    a Gestational diabetes

    b Stroke

    c Endometrial cancer

    d Cervical cancer

    e Miscarriage

127 A middle-aged man presents to his GP. He is concerned that his wife has been unable to become pregnant despite regular intercourse. He is a heavy smoker and drinker. He requests semen analysis. The following are all normal with regards to semen analysis EXCEPT:

a A volume of 2–5 mL

b A sperm count of greater than 8 million per mL

c A greater than 50% progressive mobility

d A greater than 15% normal morphology

e A greater than 25% rapid progression

128 A 35-year-old woman presents to her GP. She is concerned as she has been unable to become pregnant despite regular intercourse with her partner. Her GP arranges appropriate investigations, some of which are shown below. What is the most likely diagnosis?

LH	15 IU/L
FSH	5 IU/L
Testosterone	4 nmol/L
Prolactin	300 mU/L

a Hyperprolactinaemia

b Polycystic ovarian syndrome

c Sheehan's syndrome

d Kallman's syndrome

e Uterine fibroids

129 A 55-year-old woman presents to her GP. She complains of irregular periods and palpitations. Which investigation is most likely to lead to a diagnosis?

   a FSH alone

   b LH alone

   c FSH and LH

   d Prolactin

   e Sex hormone binding globulin

130 A 54-year-old woman is currently on hormone replacement therapy. The following are all side-effects of hormone replacement therapy EXCEPT:

   a Vaginal bleeding

   b Weight loss

   c Breast tenderness

   d Nausea

   e Headaches

131 The following are all definite contraindications to hormone replacement therapy EXCEPT:

   a Endometrial cancer

   b Vaginal bleeding

   c Pulmonary embolism

   d Deep vein thrombosis

   e Cervical cancer

132 The following are all associated risks with the use of hormone replacement therapy EXCEPT:

a Breast cancer

b Bowel cancer

c Thrombosis

d Cardiovascular disease

e Endometrial cancer

133 A 26-year-old woman presents to her GP. She complains of painful intercourse and painful periods. Speculum examination reveals the presence of blue nodules. What is the most likely diagnosis?

a Endometriosis

b Cervical cancer

c Uterine fibroids

d Pelvic inflammatory disease

e Bacterial vaginosis

134 A 27-year-old woman presents to her GP. She complains of painful intercourse and painful periods. Which investigation is most likely to lead to a diagnosis?

a Transvaginal ultrasound scan

b Abdominal ultrasound scan

c Abdominal X-ray

d Laparoscopy

e Pelvic X-ray

135 A 30-year-old woman presents to her GP. She complains of painful intercourse and painful periods. Which management plan would you instigate first?

a Total abdominal hysterectomy

b Laparoscopic uterosacral nerve ablation

c Reassure

d Combined oral contraceptive pill

e Fluoxetine

136 A 65-year-old woman presents to her GP. She complains of sudden onset vaginal itching and discharge. On examination you note the presence of an ulcer on the outer aspect of her labia majora. She is referred for appropriate investigations, which demonstrate the presence of a vulval tumour less than 2 cm in diameter with no nodal involvement. According to FIGO staging what is the most likely diagnosis?

a Stage 1

b Stage 1a

c Stage 1b

d Stage 2

e Stage 3

137 A 65-year-old woman is recently diagnosed with Stage 1b vulval carcinoma. What is the next most appropriate step in management?

a Chemotherapy

b Radiotherapy

c Reassure

d Surgery alone

e Surgery and lymphadenectomy

138 A middle-aged woman presents to her GP complaining of new onset vaginal discharge. Speculum examination reveals the presence of an erythematous raw-looking cervix. Current medication includes the oral contraceptive pill. What is the most likely diagnosis?

a Cervical polyp

b Cervical cancer

c Cervical ectropion

d Bacterial vaginosis

e Chlamydia

139 The following are all true with regards to cervical screening EXCEPT:

a In the UK, women between the age of 25 and 49 are screened three-yearly

b In the UK, women between the age of 50 and 64 are screened five-yearly

c A smear is best taken at the end of the menstrual cycle

d The screening process is non-diagnostic for cancer

e In the UK, non-sexually-active women are invited for cervical screening

140 A middle-aged woman attends a follow-up appointment with her GP following a cervical smear. The report states that there is evidence of moderate dyskaryosis. Which management plan would you instigate first?

   a Chemotherapy

   b Colposcopy

   c Reassure

   d Repeat in six weeks

   e Radiotherapy

141 A middle-aged woman presents to her GP for the results of her recent smear test. The report states there is evidence of differentiation in the upper third of the epithelium with mitotic figures in the basal two-thirds. Which management plan would you instigate first?

   a Repeat in six weeks

   b Laser vaporization

   c Diathermy

   d Excision

   e Cryocautery

142 A 63-year-old woman presents to her GP. She complains of sudden onset bleeding vaginally and a purulent discharge. She is postmenopausal. Speculum examination reveals the presence of an ulcerated cervix. What is the most likely diagnosis?

   a Cervical polyp

   b Cervical cancer

   c Cervical ectropion

   d Candida

   e Chlamydia

143 A 64-year-old woman is referred for investigation following a suspected diagnosis of cervical cancer. Following appropriate investigations a cervical carcinoma is confirmed involving the vagina but not the lower third segment. According to FIGO staging, what is the most likely diagnosis?

a Stage 1

b Stage 1a

c Stage 2

d Stage 3

e Stage 4

144 A 65-year-old woman is informed by her GP of a diagnosis of cervical carcinoma, which has spread to the lower third of her vagina. She has a past medical history of chronic obstructive pulmonary disease (COPD) and ischaemic heart disease. Which management plan would you instigate first?

a Reassure

b Urgent chemotherapy

c Urgent surgery

d Urgent radiotherapy

e Repeat biopsy in two weeks

145 A 30-year-old Afro-Caribbean woman presents to her GP. She complains of increasingly heavy periods and abdominal discomfort. What is the next most appropriate step in management?

a Reassure

b GnRH analogue

c Combined oral contraceptive pill

d Total abdominal hysterectomy

e Chemotherapy

146 A 40-year-old woman presents to her GP. She complains of irregular bleeding, which can be heavy at times. The GP refers her for appropriate tests as he suspects endometrial cancer. The investigations confirm the presence of a carcinoma confined to the uterus and cervix. According to FIGO staging, what is the most likely diagnosis?

a Stage 1

b Stage 2

c Stage 3a

d Stage 3b

e Stage 4a

147 A middle-aged woman is recently diagnosed with endometrial cancer. Investigations confirm the cancer is confined to the uterus, more specifically, the inner half of the myometrium. Which management plan would you instigate first?

   a Total abdominal hysterectomy with bilateral salpingo-oophorectomy

   b Chemotherapy

   c Radiotherapy

   d Repeat biopsy in two weeks

   e Reassure

148 Which of the following is an example of an ovarian tumour that accounts for over 50% of all ovarian malignancies?

   a Serous cystadenoma

   b Mucinous cystadenoma

   c Endometrioid carcinoma

   d Clear cell carcinoma

   e Teratoma

149 Which of the following is an example of an ovarian tumour that can contain tissue from germs cells of the ovary, hair and teeth?

   a Serous cystadenoma

   b Mucinous cystadenoma

   c Endometrioid carcinoma

   d Clear cell carcinoma

   e Teratoma

150 A woman presents to A&E. She complains of shortness of breath and abdominal discomfort. A chest X-ray confirms evidence of a right-sided pleural effusion with no evidence of collapse or consolidation. An abdominal ultrasound scan confirms evidence of an ovarian mass, which appears benign. She is a non-smoker and has no significant past medical or surgical history. What is the most likely diagnosis?

    a Serous cystadenoma

    b Mucinous cystadenoma

    c Fibroma

    d Clear cell carcinoma

    e Teratoma

151 Which of the following is an example of a slow growing, commonly malignant ovarian tumour that secretes oestrogen?

    a Serous cystadenoma

    b Mucinous cystadenoma

    c Fibroma

    d Clear cell carcinoma

    e Granulosa cell tumour

152 Which of the following is an example of a benign ovarian tumour that secretes oestrogen?

    a Serous cystadenoma

    b Mucinous cystadenoma

    c Thecoma

    d Clear cell carcinoma

    e Granulosa cell tumour

153 Which of the following is an example of a malignant tumour that has a poor prognosis and accounts for approximately 10% of all ovarian cancers?

a Serous cystadenoma

b Mucinous cystadenoma

c Thecoma

d Clear cell carcinoma

e Granulosa cell tumour

154 An elderly woman presents to her GP complaining of abdominal discomfort. She also comments that her trousers and skirts feel looser than normal. She has never had a child and is known to have had an early menarche. Which serum investigation is most likely to lead to a diagnosis?

a AFP

b βhCG

c Cancer antigen (CA) 125

d CA 19–9

e Carcinoembryonic antigen (CEA)

155 Which gene is most strongly associated with the development of ovarian carcinoma?

a *NOD 2*

b *BRCA 1*

c *p53*

d *BRCA 4*

e *BRCA 6*

156 A 70-year-old woman presents to her GP. She complains of abdominal discomfort and vaginal bleeding. She has a positive family history of ovarian cancer. What is the next most appropriate initial investigation?

   a Abdominal X-ray

   b Vaginal swab

   c Endocervical swab

   d Abdominal ultrasound scan

   e Pelvic X-ray

157 An elderly woman is recently diagnosed with ovarian cancer. Following appropriate investigations she is informed that the tumour has spread to the fallopian tubes. According to FIGO staging, what is the most likely diagnosis?

   a Stage 1a

   b Stage 1b

   c Stage 1c

   d Stage 2a

   e Stage 3

158 An elderly woman is recently diagnosed with Stage 2 ovarian cancer. What is the next most appropriate step in management?

   a Chemotherapy

   b Surgery

   c Surgery and chemotherapy

   d Reassure

   e Chemotherapy and radiotherapy

159 A 57-year-old woman presents to her GP. She comments that she feels something is coming down through her vagina. She also mentions that when she coughs she accidentally passes urine. She is morbidly obese and a life-long smoker. What is the most likely diagnosis?

a Posterior vaginal wall prolapse

b Stress incontinence

c Genuine stress incontinence

d Overflow incontinence

e Anterior vaginal wall prolapse

160 An elderly woman presents to her GP. She comments that she feels as if something is coming down through her vagina. She also informs you that she has difficulty in opening her bowels. With regards to her past obstetric history she is gravida 3, para 3. What is the most likely diagnosis?

a Posterior vaginal wall prolapse

b Stress incontinence

c Genuine stress incontinence

d Overflow incontinence

e Anterior vaginal wall prolapse

161 A middle-aged woman presents to her GP complaining of accidentally passing urine when she coughs. She has three children. What is the most likely diagnosis?

    a Posterior vaginal wall prolapse

    b Stress incontinence

    c True incontinence

    d Overflow incontinence

    e Anterior vaginal wall prolapse

162 A middle-aged obese woman presents to her GP. She complains of accidentally passing small amounts of urine and feeling a sense of incomplete emptying. She has a past medical history of depression and is currently on imipramine. What is the most likely diagnosis?

    a Posterior vaginal wall prolapse

    b Stress incontinence

    c True incontinence

    d Overflow incontinence

    e Anterior vaginal wall prolapse

163 Which management plan would you instigate first in the above patient?

    a Fluid restriction

    b Weight loss

    c Pelvic floor exercises

    d Tolterodine

    e Stop imipramine

164 The following are all risks to the fetus in a pregnant mother with chicken pox EXCEPT:

   a Visual disturbances

   b Limb hypoplasia

   c Skin scarring

   d Neurological abnormalities

   e Jaundice

165 The following are all risks to the fetus in a pregnant mother with rubella EXCEPT:

   a Cataracts

   b Heart disease

   c Renal failure

   d Hepatomegaly

   e Splenomegaly

166 The following are all true with regards to toxoplasmosis infection in pregnancy EXCEPT:

   a The majority of mothers are affected in the second trimester

   b Incubation can be up to 20 days

   c It is associated with flu-like symptoms

   d Diagnosis is by serology testing

   e It can be associated with hydrocephalus in the fetus

167 The following are all true with regards to cytomegalovirus infection in pregnancy EXCEPT:

a It has an incubation period of up to 12 weeks

b It is the least common cause of congenital neurological abnormalities

c It may cause a flu-like illness

d Primary infection is confirmed by the presence of immunoglobulin M (IgM)

e It may be associated with thrombocytopenia in the fetus

168 The following are all true with regards to Group B *Streptococcus* infection in pregnancy EXCEPT:

a The infection affects roughly one-quarter of women in pregnancy

b Risk factors for neonatal infection include pre-term labour

c Penicillin is the treatment of choice

d Pyrexia in labour is not a risk factor for neonatal infection

e Infection is typically asymptomatic

169 The following are all true with regards to parvovirus infection EXCEPT:

a Transmission occurs via respiratory droplets

b It has an incubation period of 40 days

c Diagnosis is made by serology testing

d It may cause myocarditis in the fetus

e It may cause anaemia in the fetus

170 A pregnant woman has been recently diagnosed with Listeria. What is the next most appropriate step in management?

a Doxycycline

b Penicillin

c Paracetamol

d Immediate delivery

e Reassure

171 Which of the following is the leading cause of death in pregnant women?

a Cardiac failure

b Stroke

c Venous thromboembolism

d Renal failure

e Anaemia

172 A middle-aged woman presents to her GP complaining of a new lesion on her vagina. On examination you note a pustular like lesion on her vagina, which is not painful on palpation. She has recently returned from Africa and had several episodes of unprotected intercourse. What is the most likely diagnosis?

a Chlamydia

b Gonorrhoea

c Lymphogranuloma venereum

d Donovaniasis

e Chancroid

173 What is the next most appropriate step in management for the above patient?

    a Doxycycline

    b Penicillin

    c Paracetamol

    d Excision

    e Reassure

Extended matching questions

Theme: Contraception

a Mirena coil

b Combined oral contraceptive pill

c Progesterone-only pill

d Copper coil

e Male condom

f Diaphragm

g Implant

h Female condom

i Cap

j Medroxyprogesterone IM

For each scenario described below, choose the single most appropriate answer from the above list of options. Each option may be used once, more than once or not at all.

1   Associated with an increased risk of actinomycosis and pelvic inflammatory disease.

2 Specifically contraindicated in women over the age of 35 who smoke, with a history of hypertension.

3 Associated with a reduced incidence of pelvic inflammatory disease. It is known to cause irregular bleeding in the first three months.

4 Side-effects include weight gain, irregular bleeding and an increased risk of osteoporosis.

5 Known to be an effective treatment against pelvic inflammatory disease and endometrial cancer.

Theme: Tumours

a Vulval

b Endometrial

c Ovarian

d Cervical

e Serous cystadenoma

f Clear cell

g Endometrioid

h Mucinous cystadenoma

i Teratoma

j Dysgerminoma

For each scenario described below, choose the single most appropriate answer from the above list of options. Each option may be used once, more than once or not at all.

1 Associated with an elevated serum CA 125.

2 Known to contain tissue from the germ cells of the ovary, hair and teeth.

3 The second most common malignancy in women worldwide.

4 An oestrogen-secreting tumour associated with abdominal bleeding seen commonly in women over the age of 40.

5 A malignant tumour accounting for approximately 10% of ovarian cancers that carries a poor prognosis.

Theme: Investigations

a Ultrasound scan

b High vaginal swab

c Endocervical swab

d Blood cultures

e LH:FSH ratio

f Thyroid function tests

g Prolactin

h Progesterone

i Oestrogen

j Abdominal X-ray

For each scenario described below, choose the single most appropriate answer from the above list of options. Each option may be used once, more than once or not at all.

1 The diagnostic test for gonorrhoea.

2 The diagnostic test for a woman presenting with a curd-like grey-coloured vaginal discharge.

3 A serum investigation for a middle-aged woman presenting with weight gain, acne and hirsutism.

4 An Afro-Caribbean woman presenting with painful periods and urinary retention.

5 A woman presenting with a frothy yellow discharge and strawberry-red cervix following speculum assessment.

Theme: Treatment

a Surgery

b Chemotherapy

c Radiotherapy

d Combined oral contraceptive pill

e GnRH analogues

f Mefenamic acid

g Fentanyl patch

h Surgery and chemotherapy

i Fluoxetine

j Risperidone

1 A middle-aged woman presenting with abdominal discomfort and low mood prior to commencing her period.

2 A woman continually presenting with pelvic pain two days before each period.

3 A woman recently diagnosed with stage 3 cervical cancer.

4 A woman recently diagnosed with stage 4 ovarian cancer.

5 A 25-year-old non-smoker presenting with heavy periods allergic to non-steroidal anti inflammatory drugs. She has no known past medical history.

Theme: Side-effects

a Thrombosis

b Osteoporosis

c Actinomycosis

d Ectopic pregnancy

e Weight gain

f Irregular bleeding

g Nausea

h Breast tenderness

i Acne

j Pelvic inflammatory disease

For each scenario described below, choose the single most appropriate answer from the above list of options. Each option may be used once, more than once or not at all.

1   A common side-effect of the copper coil if pregnancy occurs.

2   A serious side-effect of the combined oral contraceptive pill.

3   Associated with long-term use of medroxyprogesterone acetate injections.

4   Seen commonly with the use of the cooper coil and progesterone-only pill.

5   Associated commonly with the use of the Mirena coil within the first three months.

Theme: Sexually transmitted infections

a   Chlamydia

b   Gonorrhoea

c   Trichomonas

d   Herpes

e   Warts

f   Molluscum contagiosum

g   Crabs

h   Syphilis

i   Hepatitis B

j   Bacterial vaginosis

For each scenario described below, choose the single most appropriate answer from the above list of options. Each option may be used once, more than once or not at all.

1   Associated with a thin cream-coloured discharge and a vaginal fluid pH of greater than 4.5.

2   Associated with a wart lesion peri-anally two years post-infection.

3   Associated with multiple pearl-white lesions on the genitalia.

4   A common infection in those under the age of 25 on the combined oral contraceptive pill. It is associated with irregular vaginal bleeding and painful intercourse.

5   Associated with a frothy yellow discharge and a strawberry-red cervix.

Theme: The menstrual cycle

a Prolactin

b Oestrogen

c Progesterone

d GnRH

e FSH

f LH

g Follicular phase

h Luteal phase

i Proliferative phase

j Secretory phase

For each scenario described below, choose the single most appropriate answer from the above list of options. Each option may be used once, more than once or not at all.

1 A hormone produced by the hypothalamus and involved in the release of FSH and LH.

2 A reduction in this hormone triggers menstruation.

3 These hormones are both released during the luteal phase.

4 This hormone is directly responsible for the growth and thickening of the endometrium.

5 These hormones are released from the anterior pituitary in a pulsatile fashion.

Theme: Disorders of pregnancy I

a   Ectopic pregnancy

b   Placenta praevia

c   Placenta abruption

d   Threatened miscarriage

e   Inevitable miscarriage

f   Incomplete miscarriage

g   Complete miscarriage

h   Pre-eclampsia

i   Gestational diabetes mellitus

j   Breech presentation

For each scenario described below, choose the single most appropriate answer from the above list of options. Each option may be used once, more than once or not at all.

1   Associated with headaches or visual disturbances and known to affect obese hypertensive pregnant women.

2   Associated with fresh red vaginal bleeding in women with a gestational period of more than 24 weeks.

3   A middle-aged woman currently 20 weeks pregnant presenting with vaginal bleeding. Speculum examination reveals an undilated cervix.

4   A 23-year-old woman currently 22 weeks pregnant presenting with vaginal bleeding without passage of products of conception. Speculum examination reveals an open cervical os.

5 A pregnant woman presenting with abdominal pain and dark vaginal bleeding. A transvaginal ultrasound confirms the presence of the fetus within the fallopian tubes.

Theme: Disorders of pregnancy II

a Chicken pox

b Rubella

c Toxoplasmosis

d *Salmonella*

e Cytomegalovirus

f Parvovirus

g Listeria

h HIV

i Group B *Streptococcus*

j Bacterial vaginosis

For each scenario described below, choose the single most appropriate answer from the above list of options. Each option may be used once, more than once or not at all.

1 Present in approximately 10–12% of all pregnant women in the UK and associated with a fishy vaginal odour.

2 Known to cause fever, headaches and conjunctivitis in pregnant women following consumption of infected soft cheese.

3 Known to cause a glandular fever type of illness in pregnant women following consumption of infected meat, fruit or vegetables.

4 Associated with a flu-like illness and a fine macular rash over the trunk. Diagnosis is predominantly made through serology antibody testing.

5 A gram negative bacterial infection common in pregnancy, associated with severe vomiting and dehydration.

Theme: Physiology of pregnancy

a Cardiac output

b Ventilation rate

c Blood pressure

d Folate

e Iron

f Renal plasma flow

g Serum protein

h Red cell mass

i Serum B12

j Creatinine clearance

For each scenario described below, choose the single most appropriate answer from the above list of options. Each option may be used once, more than once or not at all.

1 Associated with a 40% increase during pregnancy.

2 Associated with an approximately 60–80% increase during pregnancy.

3 Associated with a 50% increase during pregnancy.

4 Associated with a three-fold increase in pregnancy.

5 Associated with a 10- to 20-fold increase in pregnancy.

Answers

Single best answer

1   d

The most likely time frame for conception is typically six days prior to ovulation, which corresponds to day 8–14 in an average 28-day cycle.

2   e

Cystic fibrosis is not a recognised fetal complication associated with smoking in pregnancy.

3   d

Alcohol consumption during pregnancy is associated with a lower birth weight.

4   c

Liver contains large quantities of vitamin A, which is associated with congenital abnormalities.

5   d

400 micrograms is the recommended dose and should be taken 12 weeks prior to conception until 12 weeks gestation.

6   a

Paracetamol is safe in pregnancy. Beta blockers are associated with growth restriction. Warfarin is associated with congenital abnormalities. Anti-inflammatory drugs, such as diclofenac, are linked to miscarriage in the first trimester and diuretics are known to be teratogenic.

7   a

The recognised serum markers comprising the triple test for Down's syndrome.

8   d

The ultrasound scan involves measuring the thickness of the fold of skin over the back of the fetus' neck, the baby's size and combining this with the mother's age and gestation.

9   e

This procedure involves the introduction of a needle into the uterus and withdrawing a few mL of amniotic fluid. Results are usually available within one to two weeks.

10   a

The risk of miscarriage is minimal.

11   c

This involves taking a biopsy of the placenta under ultrasound for analysis. It carries a risk of miscarriage of approximately 1%.

12   b

Oligohydramnios is typically detected between 18 and 24 weeks.

13   e

Fetal position is typically assessed after 36 weeks.

14   e

Pregnancy is associated with delayed gastric emptying and delayed lower gastrointestinal transit.

15   d

βhCG secreted by the placenta is responsible for nausea and vomiting in pregnancy.

16   b

Serum protein falls in pregnancy due to a fall in serum albumin concentration.

17   b

A common disorder in pregnancy. Risk factors include primiparity, multiple pregnancy, obesity, diabetes and chronic hypertension.

18   e

Obesity is a risk factor for pre-eclampsia.

19   a

A very low platelet count is a worrying sign and may be indicative of HELLP syndrome.

20   c

First-line management in terms of blood pressure control is methyl-dopa usually at a dose of 250 mg three times a day.

21 b

This is worrying. The patient has a low haemoglobin and platelet count. Biochemistry is likely to reveal elevated liver enzymes which would signify HELLP syndrome. At this stage immediate delivery is necessary as this is the only true cure for pre-eclampsia.

22 e

Placental abruption is a common complication of pre-eclampsia.

23 a

Placenta praevia is diagnosed typically by fresh red blood and is typically painless.

24 b

Classic description of placental abruption. Such a condition is associated with dark red blood, abdominal pain and a 'woody' uterus due to spontaneous uterine contractions.

25 a

A high fetal head or malpresentation is suggestive of placenta praevia. Her symptoms also imply the diagnosis due to a lack of abdominal pain.

26 b

This is a likely diagnosis of placenta praevia. The gold standard investigation is an ultrasound scan.

27 e

This is most definitely worrying. A significant antepartum haemorrhage resulting in hypovolaemic shock. The most appropriate step in management would therefore be aggressive fluid resuscitation.

28 d

Alcohol is not a recognised risk factor with regard to placental abruption.

29 a

This is diagnostic of placenta praevia. As the patient is haemodynamically stable and has reached term, the most appropriate management step would be delivery by caesarean section.

30 c

The WHO guidelines state that a two-hour venous glucose greater than 11 mmol/L is diagnostic of gestational diabetes mellitus.

31 d

Polyhydramnios is an associated risk in a diabetic pregnancy.

32 e

Shoulder dystocia is not a recognised complication of obstetric cholestasis.

33 b

A breech presentation is where the fetal buttocks occupy the lower uterine segment. An extended breech is associated with the fetal head in the midline.

34 a

This is a breech presentation. External cephalic version allows manipulation of the lie of the fetus into a cephalic presentation.

35   e

An increasing maternal age is associated with multiple pregnancy.

36   b

Renal failure is not a recognised complication of multiple pregnancy.

37   e

Shoulder dystocia is not a recognised fetal complication of multiple pregnancy.

38   b

The first stage of labour is associated with cervical dilatation. The second stage is the time interval from full dilation to fetal delivery.

39   c

Internal rotation involves rotation from a lower occipital transverse position to an occipito anterior position.

40   d

The uterus is prone to rupture in a multiparous labour.

41   b

Fetal heart auscultation should occur typically every 15 minutes and be performed for a 1-minute duration.

42   b

A fetal bradycardia is typically less than 110 beats per minute.

43 a

Syntometrine is the oxytocic drug of choice in labour but is contraindicated in women with hypertension, asthma and active cardiac disease.

44 e

Additional indications include diabetes mellitus.

45 e

Such a scoring system comprises of the following parameters: cervical dilatation, effacement, consistency, position and fetal station. The highest possible score is 13.

46 c

The maternal bladder should ideally be empty prior to operative delivery.

47 c

Ventouse delivery requires a minimal force to be applied.

48 e

There is failure of progression of the first stage of labour and this is an indication for immediate caesarean section.

49 b

In pre-term labour, steroids help to promote lung maturity. Salbutamol helps to inhibit uterine smooth muscle contractility.

50   a

This patient is suffering from mastitis. The most common offending organism is *Staphylococcus aureus*. Additional organisms include *Staphylococcus epidermidis* and *Streptococci*.

51   b

Flucloxacillin or erythromycin are suitable antibiotics of choice.

52   a

Retained products of conception predisposes oneself to sepsis and hence antibiotic cover is essential.

53   d

The gold standard investigation in such a scenario.

54   e

The criteria of the Apgar score include skin colour, pulse rate, reflex irritability, muscle tone and breathing. A score of 7–10 is generally normal.

55   d

Classic presentation of shoulder dystocia, which carries a current incidence rate of approximately 0.5%.

56   e

Excess maternal weight is a risk factor for shoulder dystocia.

57   d

Primary post partum haemorrhage is associated with polyhydramnios.

58 b

The combined oral contraceptive pill is an excellent form of contraception in this age group, particularly in those who suffer from menorrhagia.

59 b

Contraindications to the use of the combined oral contraceptive pill are pregnancy, hypertension, migraine, thrombosis, ischaemic heart disease, stroke, liver disease and smokers over 35 years of age.

60 c

The reason why a barrier method of contraception should be used for this length is that it takes approximately seven days of pill usage to suppress ovarian activity and hence there is a risk of conception without the use of a barrier method.

61 e

Due to her history of hypertension and life-long smoking, the combined oral contraceptive pill is specifically contraindicated. The implant device has been shown to reduce the risk of pelvic inflammatory disease and endometrial cancer.

62 b

The combined oral contraceptive pill is associated with thrombosis, hypertension and migraine in the main.

63 e

The implant device would be most suitable due to her history of hypertension, questionable compliance with oral medication and past history of pelvic inflammatory disease.

64   d

Long-term use of medroxyprogesterone IM has been linked to osteoporosis.

65   e

The Mirena coil is associated with a reduced risk of ectopic pregnancy as well as pelvic inflammatory disease.

66   c

The copper coil has been specifically linked to menorrhagia and an increased risk of pelvic inflammatory disease.

67   b

The levonorgestrel pill is recommended at a dose of 1.5 mg.

68   a

An endocervical swab is the gold standard diagnostic test for gonorrhoea.

69   a

Alternative options include doxycycline or erythromycin.

70   c

Classical presentation of trichomonas infection. Diagnosis is typically via a high vaginal swab.

71   e

The drug of choice in trichomonas infection at a dose of 2 g orally.

72   e

This patient is most likely to be suffering from genital herpes and a swab from the lesion base is often diagnostic.

73   c

This patient is most likely to be suffering from genital herpes. Aciclovir is the treatment of choice.

74   a

A classic presentation of genital warts. Alternative treatment options include cryotherapy, excision or laser treatment.

75   a

Primary syphilis is diagnosed by the presence of a single painless genital ulcer, commonly referred to as a chancre.

76   b

A spirochaete with an incubation period of up to 90 days.

77   b

Such wart-like lesions are known as condylomata lata. Secondary syphilis occurs usually within two years of infection.

78   e

This patient is suffering from syphilis. Treatment of choice is procaine penicillin IM or doxycycline if penicillin allergic.

79   c

Chlamydial infection is common under the age of 25. Complications of such an infection include pelvic inflammatory disease, infertility and ectopic pregnancy.

80   a

Such an infection is common in diabetics, pregnancy and post-anti-biotic usage.

81   a

Alternative treatments include nystatin or econazole.

82   d

Clue cells are diagnostic of Bacterial vaginosis.

83   e

Additional organisms include *Mycoplasma hominis* and *Mobiluncus* species.

84   e

Additional complications include fetal growth restriction and low birth weight.

85   e

The organism typically affects the endocervix, urethra, rectum and eyes.

86   a

This patient is suffering from candida infection. A high vaginal swab is diagnostic.

87   a

Pearl-white lesions are characteristic of molluscum contagiosum. Cryotherapy is the treatment of choice.

88   d

The brown specks are most likely louse droppings, which indicate crab infection. Treatment usually involves topical malathion.

89   e

Bacterial vaginosis does not present with irregular bleeding.

90   a

The Pearl index is defined as the number of women who will become pregnant if 100 women use that form of contraception for one year. The Pearl index associated with male sterilization is 0.05.

91   d

The combined oral contraceptive pill is in fact a useful treatment for menorrhagia.

92   b

The progesterone-only pill is associated with weight gain, not loss.

93   c

Renal failure is not a recognised contraindication to the use of the Mirena coil. Additional contraindications include endometrial carcinoma.

94 e

Additional contraindications include ectopic pregnancy and copper allergy.

95 d

Malignancy is not associated with having a vasectomy.

96 d

A miscarriage is defined as the involuntary loss of pregnancy prior to 24 weeks gestation. An inevitable miscarriage is associated without the passage of products of conception.

97 e

In this case the fetus is still viable and only 25% are likely to miscarry.

98 b

A transvaginal ultrasound scan is the gold standard investigation for a suspected miscarriage.

99 b

This method is effective up to 9 weeks gestation and does not require anaesthesia. Cervical dilatation is typically performed after 12 weeks gestation.

100 d

The partner has no rights with regards to abortion according to the 1967 Abortion Act.

101 b

In the first trimester, polycystic ovaries are most strongly associated with recurrent miscarriage.

102 d

A serum βhCG of greater than 1500 IU is strongly suggestive of an ectopic in addition to the patient's symptoms.

103 c

These are the gold standard investigations for a suspected ectopic pregnancy.

104 e

Other less common sites of implantation include the cornua of the uterus, cervix, ovary or abdominal cavity.

105 b

Previous pelvic inflammatory disease is associated with a 10-fold risk of ectopic pregnancy.

106 e

This hormone is released from the hypothalamus and stimulates the release of FSH and LH.

107 b

LH stimulates ovulation and is responsible for the development of the corpus luteum.

108 e

These hormones are produced by the corpus luteum until it disintegrates after approximately 9–11 days.

109 d

This occurs specifically during the proliferative phase of the cycle.

110 d

This all helps to prepare for a fertilized ovum.

111 d

The average loss of blood is typically 30 mL.

112 e

Menstruation itself involves arterial constriction of the endometrium and subsequent necrosis.

113 a

Iron deficiency anaemia is classical of menorrhagia and is detected by the presence of pencil cells on the blood film.

114 c

An alternative form of treatment would be the combined oral contraceptive pill but would be unsuitable here due to the presence of hypertension and smoking history.

115 d

The Mirena coil is associated with irregular bleeding within the first three months of usage.

116 e

Endometrial cancer may occur but is certainly not a common complication of the procedure.

117 b

This patient is experiencing dysmenorrhoea. Anti-inflammatory drugs such as mefenamic acid are the mainstay form of treatment.

118 a

Classical features of Turner's syndrome.

119 d

This patient is suffering from premenstrual syndrome. Selective serotonin reuptake inhibitors such as fluoxetine have been proven to be beneficial in terms of symptom control.

120 c

This patient has suffered an ectopic pregnancy and is haemodynamically unstable. An urgent laparoscopy is therefore needed.

121 a

Additional symptoms would include obesity and male pattern baldness.

122 d

This patient is suffering from polycystic ovarian syndrome. An abdominal ultrasound scan is the gold standard investigation of choice.

123 d

This patient is suffering from polycystic ovarian syndrome. An LH:FSH ratio is the most appropriate serum investigation.

124 c

This patient has polycystic ovarian syndrome. The combined oral contraceptive pill helps to regulate periods, hirsutism and acne.

125 c

Serum FSH is usually normal in patients with polycystic ovarian syndrome.

126 d

The only associated malignancy with polycystic ovarian syndrome is endometrial cancer.

127 b

A sperm count greater than 20 million per mL is deemed normal.

128 b

This patient has a raised LH:FSH ratio, a normal prolactin and a raised testosterone concentration, which is in keeping with polycystic ovarian syndrome.

129 c

In view of her symptoms and age this patient is most probably experiencing menopausal changes. FSH and LH are the gold standard investigations and are both likely to be raised.

130 b

Weight gain is a common complication of hormone replacement therapy.

131 e

Endometrial cancer is a definite contraindication to the use of hormone replacement therapy.

132 b

Hormone replacement therapy in fact lowers one's risk of bowel cancer.

133 a

Endometriosis is associated with painful intercourse and periods. Vaginal endometriosis is characterised by the presence of blue nodules following speculum examination.

134 d

This patient is suffering from endometriosis. Laparoscopy is diagnostic.

135 d

This patient is most probably suffering from endometriosis. The combined oral contraceptive pill is often the first-line treatment of choice.

136 a

Further information on FIGO staging for vulval cancer is available online at: www.nci.nih.gov/cancertopics/pdq/treatment/vulvar/HealthProfessional/page4 (accessed 1 November 2009).

137 e

Stage 1a carcinoma is managed by wide local excision. All other stages are treated by wide local excision and lymphadenectomy.

138 c

Classical presentation of a cervical ectropion seen commonly during puberty, pregnancy and the use of the oral contraceptive pill.

139 c

A smear is best taken mid-cycle.

140 b

Moderate dyskaryosis is an indication for immediate colposcopy.

141 d

This is cervical intraepithelial neoplasia (CIN) 2 and is most appropriately treated via excision.

142 b

This form of cancer is the second commonest in women worldwide. Squamous cell is the most common histological type. Approximately 1 in 10 to 1 in 20 cases of cervical cancer are adenocarcinoma.

143 c

Further information on FIGO staging for cervical cancer is available online at http://screening.iarc.fr/viaviliappendix1.php (accessed 1 November 2009).

144 d

This patient has stage 3 disease. Radiotherapy is the treatment of choice for stages 2b or greater.

145 b

This patient is suffering from uterine fibroids, a common tumour affecting Afro-Caribbean women. GnRH analogues or progesterone tablets are the mainstay form of medical management and should be trialled before surgery.

146 b

Further information on FIGO staging for endometrial cancer is available online at: www.cancer.org/docroot/CRI/content/CRI_2_4 _3X_How_is_endometrial_cancer_staged.asp?sitearea (accessed 1 November 2009).

147 a

This is stage 1b endometrial cancer. Such surgery is the mainstay form of treatment for stage 1 or stage 2 disease.

148 a

This tumour may be benign or malignant in nature.

149 e

They are usually quite small but may cause pain once ruptured.

150 c

Fibromas are ovarian tumours associated with a pleural effusion and ascites, commonly referred to as Meig's syndrome.

151 e

Such tumours may cause post-menopausal bleeding or endometrial carcinoma.

152 c

Such tumours are similar to granulosa cell tumours.

153 d

Classical description of a clear cell carcinoma.

154 c

This patient is most likely to be suffering from ovarian cancer in view of her weight loss and abdominal pain. Early menarche is a risk factor for such a cancer and serum CA 125 is often raised in the vast majority.

155 b

BRCA 1 and *BRCA 2* are linked to the development of ovarian cancer.

156 d

It is likely that this patient is suffering from ovarian cancer in view of her symptoms and positive family history. An abdominal ultrasound scan is diagnostic.

157 d

Further information on FIGO staging for ovarian cancer is available online at: http://ovariancancer.about.com/od/testsdiagnosis/a/FIGO_stages.htm (accessed 1 November 2009).

158 c

Surgery with chemotherapy is the treatment of choice in all patients except those with stage 1a tumours.

159 e

Anterior vaginal wall prolapse is often associated with urinary symptoms during episodes of increased abdominal pressure, such as coughing.

160 a

Posterior vaginal wall prolapse is associated with a difficulty in defecation. Childbirth is a recognised cause of prolapse.

161 b

Classical description of stress incontinence.

162 d

Imipramine is a tricyclic antidepressant and is associated with urinary retention and overflow incontinence due to detrusor dysfunction.

163 e

Imipramine should be stopped initially, due to its anticholinergic side-effects.

164 e

Jaundice is not a recognised fetal risk associated with maternal chicken pox.

165 c

Renal failure is not a recognised fetal risk associated with maternal rubella infection.

166 a

The majority of mothers are affected in the third trimester of pregnancy.

167 c

It is in fact the most common cause of neurological congenital abnormalities.

168 d

Pyrexia in labour is a recognised risk factor for neonatal infection.

169 b

Parvovirus has an incubation period of approximately 18–20 days.

170 b

Penicillin is the treatment of choice. Diagnosis is made by blood cultures.

171 c

It has an incidence of roughly 65 per 100 000 per year in pregnant women.

172 c

The infection may also affect the vulva or cervix.

173 a

The usual dose is 100 mg twice daily for three weeks.

Extended matching questions

Theme: Contraception

1 d

The copper coil is also associated with a risk of perforation.

2 b

Additional contraindications include stroke, ischaemic heart disease and liver disease.

3 a

The Mirena coil may also cause an increased risk of ovarian cysts and perforation.

4 j

Osteoporosis is only seen in those following long-term use of medroxyprogesterone IM.

5 g

The implant device can also be used during breastfeeding.

Theme: Tumours

1   c

An elevated serum CA 125 is diagnostic of ovarian cancer.

2   i

Teratomas are typically benign and rarely undergo malignant change.

3   d

Breast cancer is the most common malignancy in women.

4   b

Such tumours are seen commonly in obese women as adipose tissue increases the levels of oestrogen significantly.

5   f

Classical description of a clear cell carcinoma.

Theme: Investigations

1 c

Treatment is via ciprofloxacin or ampicillin.

2 b

This is most likely to be candida infection, which is most appropriately diagnosed via a high vaginal swab.

3 e

This is a presentation of polycystic ovarian syndrome. The LH:FSH ratio is diagnostic and is usually raised.

4 a

A presentation of fibroids, which is common in the Afro-Caribbean population.

5 b

This is a clinical presentation of trichomonas, most appropriately diagnosed by a high vaginal swab.

Theme: Treatment

1 i

This patient is experiencing premenstrual syndrome. Selective serotonin reuptake inhibitors such as fluoxetine have been proven to be beneficial.

2 f

Classical dysmenorrhoea, which is most appropriately treated with anti-inflammatory drugs such as mefenamic acid.

3 c

Radiotherapy is the treatment of choice for stage 2b and above cervical cancer.

4 h

Surgery and chemotherapy is the mainstay form of treatment in all patients with ovarian cancer except those with stage 1a.

5 d

The combined oral contraceptive pill is an excellent choice of treatment for menorrhagia.

Theme: Side-effects

1   d

Ectopic pregnancy is a recognised complication of the copper coil.

2   a

Additional serious side-effects include hypertension and migraine.

3   b

A well-documented side-effect of long-term use.

4   d

Both are linked with an increased risk of ectopic pregnancy.

5   f

Irregular bleeding is a well-documented side-effect of the Mirena coil within the first three months.

Theme: Sexually transmitted infections

1   j

Other diagnostic criteria include the presence of clue cells on microscopy.

2   h

More specifically secondary syphilis caused by *Treponema pallidum* infection.

3   f

Such infection is typically caused by a pox virus. Treatment involves cryotherapy.

4   a

Treatment typically involves azithromycin or doxycycline.

5   c

Classical presentation of trichomonas infection. Metronidazole is the treatment of choice.

Theme: The menstrual cycle

1   d

Such hormones are released by the anterior pituitary in a pulsatile fashion.

2   c

Menstruation comprises arterial constriction and subsequent endometrial necrosis.

3   b and c

Such hormones are released by the corpus luteum.

4   b

This is commonly referred to as the proliferative phase of the menstrual cycle.

5   e and f

GnRH from the hypothalamus triggers their release.

Theme: Disorders of pregnancy I

1   h

Classical presentation of pre-eclampsia. The ultimate cure is fetal delivery.

2   b

Such patients tend not to experience any form of abdominal pain or discomfort.

3   d

Classical description of a threatened miscarriage.

4   e

An open os is diagnostic of an inevitable miscarriage. There is no associated passage of products of conception.

5   a

The fallopian tubes are the most common sites of implantation in an ectopic pregnancy.

Theme: Disorders of pregnancy II

1 j

Bacterial vaginosis can often present with a cream-coloured discharge as well.

2 g

Fetal infection may result in miscarriage, stillbirth and pre-term delivery.

3 c

Diagnosis is by serology testing and treatment with spiramycin is beneficial.

4 b

The fetus may suffer from cataracts, deafness, learning difficulties and congenital heart disease.

5 d

Such a bacterium may be contracted from ingestion of contaminated meat or eggs.

Theme: Physiology of pregnancy

1   a

The increase is due to a fall in vascular resistance.

2   f

The glomerular filtration rate also subsequently increases.

3   j

This results in a fall in serum urea and creatinine.

4   e

This is due to an increased blood volume in pregnancy, increased fetal needs and blood loss during delivery.

5   d

This is due to increased fetal needs and red cell development.

Index

Page numbers to questions (Q) and answers (A) are given in the following format Q/A